Studies in Tibetan Medicine

Studies in Tibetan Medicine

Elisabeth Finckh, M.D.

Snow Lion Publications
Ithaca, New York USA

Snow Lion Publications
P.O. Box 6483
Ithaca, New York 14851
USA

First Edition USA 1988

Printed in USA

Library of Congress Catalog Number

ISBN 0-937938-61-0

Library of Congress Cataloging-in-Publication Data

Finckh, Elisabeth.
Studies in Tibetan medicine / Elisabeth Finckh. — 1st ed. USA.
p. cm.
Bibliography: p.
Includes index.
ISBN 0-937938-61-0 : $14.95
1. Medicine—Tibetan. I. Title.
R603.T5F57 1988
610'.9515—dc 19
88-39158
CIP

Contents

Theory and Practice

THEORY OF TIBETAN MEDICINE

Tibetan medicine, which certainly has its own distinctive character, is so multifarious that it would be impossible to cover this complex topic completely in such a short paper. The following principles formed the basis for the research into the theoretical foundations of Tibetan medicine.

Oral instruction by Tibetan doctors. By way of introduction I should like to mention that I am a specialist in internal medicine and have also been trained in neurology, psychiatry and tropical medicine. For twenty-five years now I have been studying and also practicing Asian methods of treatment. My interest in Tibet began when I was young, and it was a pure and simple curiosity to learn more about a topic on which hardly any books existed which led me to grasp the first available opportunity to get into contact with Tibetan doctors after political developments in Tibet had made this possible. In 1962 I went to the Himalayas for three months to search for the Tibetan doctors who had just set up a medical school in Dharamsala. I was able to study there with the support of His Holiness the Dalai Lama, who granted me a long private audience and directed his personal physician, Yeshe Donden, to explain everything to me. The course of study was very arduous because my knowledge of the Tibetan language proved to be inadequate. However I did come to realize that Western doctors will never be able to understand Tibetan medicine, to them a totally unfamiliar field, without oral instruction by Tibetan doctors.

Medical terminology. When acupuncture, another Asian method of healing was introduced in the West—and it has in the meantime acquired academic recognition in the universities and been tried out and put into practice—several mistakes were made: the help of Sinologists in the translations of important Chinese medical works was called in far too late; this method of healing was applied far too soon and too much time was wasted on unnecessary philosophical speculations; and finally there was, right from the start, no adequate medical terminology. These mistakes must not be repeated with Tibetan medicine. Therefore, our first step must be to establish a medical terminology which is taken from the sources available and clarified with the help and advice of Tibetan doctors and Tibetologists. It would be presumptuous for an amateur Tibetologist like myself to dare to tackle such difficult sources without the help of Tibetologists. I should like to trace briefly the developments which led up to the publication of a book (which has now appeared in English under the title *Foundations of Tibetan Medicine*) that represents a first step towards a thorough documentation of Tibetan medicine. After my first visit to Dharamsala in 1962, there followed further intensive studies, which included the improving of my knowledge of the Tibetan language, an extensive exchange of letters with my Tibetan teacher, and the collection of a great deal of material on the subject. Then in 1967 I went to Dharamsala a second time and also visited Tibetan doctors at work in other areas of the Himalayas. His Holiness the Dalai Lama again granted me a long private audience. My chief concern was to establish a medical terminology using the sources available.

Research into the sources. Tibetan doctors possess a standard work known as the *Four Treatises* (*rGyud bzhi*),[1] which must form the starting point for any study of the original sources. The medical terminology, the rules, and the system of Tibetan medicine must be derived from this book which contains 156 chapters and is written in metric form with four-line stanzas, nine syllables to a line.

Influences on Tibetan medicine. The specific character of Tibetan medicine only becomes apparent when the influences on Tibetan medicine are known: Indian and Chinese ideas especially exerted their influence on Tibetan medicine and thus it is necessary to study ancient Indian and ancient Chinese medicine. Tibetan medicine is interwoven with Buddhism and therefore a good knowledge of Buddhism, particularly Tibetan Buddhism, is vital. Above all, one should also take into account pre-Buddhist influences[2] such as the ancient Tibetan Bon-religion and shamanism.

Basic concepts. The fundamental element of Tibetan medicine is the three-part division, just as the two-part division (the Yin-Yang principle) is fundamental to Chinese medicine. If the three "principles" or "humors"—wind (*rlung*), bile (*mkhris pa*), and phlegm (*bad kan*)—remain in equilibrium, the body remains healthy. If, however, certain factors cause these three principles to become disordered, disease occurs. Thus, healing is effected by restoring the lost equilibrium and not by the symptomatic treatment of a particular organ; in other words, Tibetan medicine is a holistic therapy. The system of Tibetan medicine almost always depends upon this three-part division; diagnosis and therapy are held to be impossible without knowledge of the three humors, and this is borne out in practice. Tibetan medicine is above all a doctrine of constitution. The concept that the body with its anatomical-physiological, psychic and intellectual functions acts as a mirror of the macrocosm should be mentioned as a further important aspect. This world of analogies, of corresponding phenomena, in which fine sub-strata of non-material nature make possible an interaction of body and mind cannot be compared to our Western concepts and can hardly be explained in Western terms. We can merely observe that Tibetan medicine is primarily oriented towards *functions* and not towards material sub-strata. Unfortunately I do not have time to mention in detail here the theoretical side of Tibetan medicine, the religious background, particularly the belief in and fear of evil spirits, the influence of shamanism, healings performed according to Bon rites, means of protection against evil spirits, amulets, thread crosses, "fateful" illnesses, tutelary gods, demonic influences, and other typical aspects—all of which go towards making Tibetan medicine so colorful and multifarious. Background information on medical history must be omitted as well although medicine even played an important political role: the conversion of the Mongols to Buddhism was based to a large extent on the influence of Tibetan medicine as practiced by Tibetan monks; medicine-lamas had been summoned from Tibet to be court physicians at the courts of the Mongol princes.

PRACTICE OF TIBETAN MEDICINE

The practice of Tibetan medicine presents us with a very large field of study including diagnosis and therapy, and may be illustrated most clearly in schematic form. To this end we shall turn to the system of Tibetan medicine itself to find our bearings. This system is like a tree with three roots, nine trunks, 47 branches and 224 leaves. The leaves correspond to specific and the branches to general details. Root A, the Root of Arrangement of the parts of the body, consists of two trunks; Root B, the Root of Diagnosis, three trunks; and Root C, the Root of Therapy, four trunks. These nine trunks correspond to the nine parts of medical science, which I would like to describe briefly.

Healthy organism (= Embryology, Physiology and Anatomy—Trunk I). The first part of medical science (Embryology, Physiology and Anatomy)—like the second part (Pathology)—inserted here between the comments on Theory and those on Practice, is very important to the understanding of Tibetan medicine. We have already ascertained that Tibetan medicine is primarily oriented towards functions and not towards material sub-strata and added that we should not approach this Asian method of healing with our Western concepts. This maxim becomes obvious if we take anatomy as an example: because of the way in which burials were conducted, Tibetan doctors certainly could have taken the opportunity of undertaking detailed anatomical studies. However, no endeavor seems to have been made to discover the actual anatomical structure of the human body—on the contrary, a sort of diagram depicting all the *functions* of the body seems to have been more im-

The System

ROOTS		TRUNKS	BRANCHES	LEAVES
Root A				
Arrangement of the parts of the body	I	Healthy Organism	3	25
(*gnas lugs rtsa ba*)	II	Diseased Organism	9	63
			12	88
Root B				
Diagnosis	III	Observation	2	6
(*dngos 'dzin rtsa ba*)	IV	Palpation	3	3
	V	Questioning	3	29
			8	38
Root C				
Therapy	VI	Nutrition	6	35
(*gso ba'i rtsa ba*)	VII	Behavior	3	6
	VIII	Medicines	15	50
	IX	Methods of Treatment (external)	3	7
			27	98
Totals: 3 Roots		9 Trunks	47 Branches	224 Leaves

portant. The anatomical science developed by Tibetan doctors which is, in principle, taken from Indian medicine, does not correspond to the actual anatomy of the human body. For this reason, defining and translating the terms involved presents us with great difficulties when expressing Tibetan terms in the context of Western medicine. A particular problem concerns the fact that the "organs" of Tibetan medicine are not identical with those of Western anatomical science. The Tibetans regard their organs not only as real sub-strata but also as reflections of their functions on the surface of the body. The area of invisible forces, vibrations, currents, wheels (*'khor lo*), life-veins, etc. beyond the visible man and other such concepts are to be explained in this way. They are clearly expressed in the anatomical charts. This approach also makes it possible to see man with his organs as being in a subtle and at the same time direct, relationship to the macrocosm. Tibetan medicine is fundamentally a psycho-physical, holistic doctrine and all its therapeutic methods must be viewed bearing this aspect in mind.

Diseased organism (= Pathology—Trunk II). It would be worthwhile presenting this discipline in greater detail because although the "eight-branched knowledge" (*yan lag brgyad pa*) taken over from Indian medicine is at its heart, pathology in fact demonstrates such typically Tibetan characteristics as the division into 4 × 101 illnesses. It is also worth mentioning that in some points the Tibetan "eight-branched knowledge" is different from the Indian.

Diagnosis. The system of Tibetan medicine is also of particular importance because it illustrates the relations of the various disciplines to one another. Root A consists of two trunks with 88 specific details. Root C (Therapy) consists of four trunks with 98 specific details. However, Root B (Diagnosis) has far fewer specific details: (a) Trunk III, observation—two branches, 6 leaves; (b) Trunk IV, Palpation—three branches, three leaves and (c) Trunk V, Questioning—three branches and 29 leaves; this is a grand total of 38 leaves. Of the 224 leaves within the system, only these 38 leaves or specific details are to be found in the discipline of diagnosis. Diagnostic methods play a relatively minor part in the system (and accordingly in the practice) of Tibetan medicine. Apart from a very extensive general examination and a particularly thorough abdominal diagnosis, Tibetans use, almost exclusively, the following diagnostic methods:

(a) Examination of urine (Observation—Trunk III). I was able to study this method thoroughly both at the medical school in Dharamsala and by observing itinerant doctors at work in other regions of the Himalayas. In addition I had the oppor-

tunity of observing urinary examinations which a Tibetan doctor carried out on European patients when Yeshe Donden spent some time as a guest in my practice during his trip to Europe in 1970. The urinary examination was carried out on the basis of the three types of constitution. This diagnosis together with the two methods of examination described below was in fact very accurate. For this examination Tibetan doctors use a small clean bowl into which morning urine is poured and then stirred with a pale wooden stick. The examination of the urine takes quite a long time because the following characteristics must be studied: the formation of vapor, color, smell, the formation of bubbles and sediment. Normal, healthy urine has definite characteristics corresponding to each of the three constitutional types. If these characteristics vary, then the illness diagnosed from the urine will be present.

The examination of the tongue is also an important method of diagnosis: here as in all Tibetan diagnostic methods, the characteristics are related to the three constitutional types.

(b) Examination of pulse (Palpation—Trunk IV). In the opinion of Tibetan doctors the examination of the pulse is the most important method of diagnosis because it supplies information about the functions of the organs. The pulse diagnosis is based on the stability of the function, i.e. "The relative length of time during which a particular function can be observed as remaining constant".[3] Therefore, it is wrong to equate what we in the West understand as organs with the functional scope of Tibetan "organs." In Tibetan medicine the organs are classified into two groups as follows:

1. The five solid organs (*don*): heart (*snying*); liver (*mchin pa*); lungs (*glo ba*); spleen (*mcher pa*); and kidneys (*mkhal ma*).
2. The six hollow organs (*snod*): large intestine (*long ka*); gall bladder (*mkhris pa*); small intestine (*rgyu ma*); stomach (*pho ba*); urinary bladder (*lgang pa*); and an organ *bsam se'u*.

Tibetan doctors examine the functions of these organs at 12 points on the hands (6 on each hand). The best time of day for such an examination is early in the morning when the patient should have an empty stomach if possible. The doctor uses his right hand to examine the pulses on the left-hand side of the patient's body and his left hand for those on the right-hand side. The palpation is carried out with the index finger (*mtshon*), the middle finger (*kan ma*), and the ring finger (*chag*).

In Volume I[4] of my study I recorded the following important discovery: the Tibetan classification of the organs into solid organs (*don*) and the hollow organs (*snod*) is identical with the Chinese classification into Yin (*tsang*) and Yang (*fu*). Although the Tibetan pulse diagnosis differs from the Chinese one in a number of ways, it must in principle be of Chinese origin. Also of interest in this context are the relations among the three humors—wind (*rlung*), bile (*mkhris pa*) and phlegm (*bad kan*)—and the organs. One cannot do justice to the central significance attached to pulse diagnosis by Tibetan doctors, themselves first-rate diagnosticians using this method, merely by mentioning a few details. Nor do I have time to mention the historical context and explain in what way the Chinese and Tibetan methods of pulse diagnosis differ. In Volume Two I have devoted a particularly long chapter to pulse diagnosis because this method of examination is considered to be so important by Tibetan doctors. However I should mention that it would probably be very difficult for Western doctors to learn the art of pulse diagnosis because our sense of touch is not keen enough. From the point of view of Western medicine, the pulse diagnosis is regarded as difficult, if not impossible, to explain anyway. I was able to make some very interesting observations when Yeshe Donden examined patients in my practice whose illnesses were known to me: his pulse diagnosis was invariably very good.

(c) Anamnesis (Questioning—Trunk V). When compiling a case history, a Tibetan doctor is concerned with establishing the constitutional type of the patient because he needs to know this in order to choose the right therapy. Again, this method of examination demonstrates throughout the typical three-part division. First of all come questions of a general nature; then specifically pointed questions in order to establish and, to a

certain extent, narrow down the constitutional type of the patient concerned and the clinical picture present.

All in all, 29 questions are posed with regard to: (a) productive causes (*slong rkyen*), 3 questions; (b) conditions of illness (*na lugs*), 23 questions; and (c) (habits in connection with) food (*zas*), 3 questions. These 29 questions (making up the 29 leaves of Trunk V = Questioning of the System) are very important. It is hard to imagine that any other medical system could determine in such a precise and ingenious way and with such accuracy the constitutional type and the condition of the patient through questions; these 29 questions are indeed a typical characteristic of Tibetan medicine. This is also the reason why Tibetan doctors regard this method of diagnosis as being of such significance.

Therapy. With 98 of the 224 leaves, the Root of Therapy is the largest in the system of Tibetan medicine. The importance of this discipline within the framework of Tibetan medicine as a whole is correspondingly great. This discipline may be illustrated most effectively by means of a systematic survey because in this way the characteristic three-part division and the doctrine of constitution can be most clearly seen:

a) Trunk VI	Nutrition	6 Branches	35 Leaves
b) Trunk VII	Behavior	3 Branches	6 Leaves
c) Trunk VIII	Medicines	15 Branches	50 Leaves
d) Trunk IX	Methods of Treatment (external)	3 Branches	7 Leaves

The Root of Therapy contains 27 branches and 98 leaves.

(a) Nutrition (zas*—Trunk VI).* Here one must differentiate between: Food (*zas*) e.g. cereals and pulse, meat, oils, vegetables, etc. and Drink (*skom*) e.g. milk and milk-products (buttermilk, curds, cheese, yak milk, etc.), water (7 sorts), alcoholic drinks.

All sorts of food and drink have positive or negative effects on the three constitutional types and these effects are accurately documented. Great importance is also attached to certain dietary rules, e.g. the Tibetans are aware of many combinations of foods which do not go well together and are therefore indigestible— fish and milk, milk and fruits, poultry and curds, etc. A lot of attention is paid to correct eating habits, e.g. it is considered good to drink at the beginning and at the end of a meal.

*(b) Behavior (*spyod pa—*Trunk VII).* As far as day-time behavior is concerned, bile types should, for example, behave in a calm and restful way whereas phlegm-types should move around a lot. If phlegm-types have not had enough sleep at night, they should not try to make up for it during the day, whereas wind-types may catch up on lost sleep during the day. There are also definite rules for each constitutional type with regard to seasonal influences as well as the various climatic conditions; for example, wind-types should live in a warm climate as should phlegm-types, but bile-types are better off in a cool climate. Thus, all these rules of behavior are related to the three constitutional types and must be considered accordingly.

*(c) Medicines (*sman—*Trunk VIII).* Ninety percent of Tibetan medical literature is concerned with medicines and their classification according to origin, potency, application and qualities; herbal medicines are particularly important. The following categories of medicines are described:

Taste (*ro*). Wind: sweet (*mngar ba*); sour (*skyur ba*); saline (*lan tsha ba*). Bile: sweet (*mngar ba*); bitter (*kha ba*); astringent (*bska ba*). Phlegm: pungent (*tsha ba*); sour (*skyur ba*); astringent (*bska ba*).

Potency (*nus pa*). Wind: oily (*snum pa*); heavy (*lci ba*); smooth (*'jam pa*). Bile: cool (*bsil ba*); thin (*sla ba*); blunt (*rtul ba*). Phlegm: sharp (*rno ba*); rough (*rtsub pa*); light (*yang ba*).

There are many other classifications besides this one: the relations of medicines to the five elements, classifications, divisions into various groups, divisions according to functions, etc.

It is a good idea to present once again a systematic picture of Tibetan medicines—there is really no other way of getting to grips with this enormous field of study—in order to describe the various forms of medicines and their relations to the three constitutional types:

Sedating Medicines	(*zhi byed*)	
Soups (liquids)	(*khu ba*)	
Medicinal oils (butter)	(*sman mar*)	for Wind-types
Syrups (decoctions)	(*thang*)	
Powders	(*cur ni*)	for Bile-types
Pills	(*ril bu*)	
Pastes	(*tres sam*)	for Phlegm-types
Cleansing Medicines	(*sbyong byed*)	
Oily enemas	(*'jam rtsi*)	for Wind-types
Purgatives	(*bshal*)	for Bile-types
Emetics	(*skyug sman*)	for Phlegm-types

*(d) Methods of Treatment—external (*dpyad—*Trunk IX)*. The classification of these methods of treatment and their relations to the three constitutional types will also be presented in a systematic way:

1. Inunction with massage (*bsku mnye*)
2. Mongolian (method of) cauterization (*hor gyi me btsa'*) for Wind-types
3. Production of sweat (*rngul dbyung*)
4. Blood-letting (*gtar ga*)
5. "The magic water wheel" (a sort of hydrophatic treatment) (*chu yi 'phrul 'khor*) for Bile-types
6. Heat treatment (*dugs*)
7. Burning—moxibustion (*btsa'*) for Phlegm-types

Surgery plays a relatively minor role; operations are only performed if there is no other possibility of healing the patient. Blood transfusions are also regarded with a good deal of skepticism. However, Tibetan doctors do know a lot about treating dislocations and sprains. I frequently had the opportunity of admiring the skill of these doctors in treating even serious dislocations and fractures in adults and especially in children. In addition to the above mentioned methods of treatment which have been described systematically, there are also a great number of others common to Tibetan medicine.

Applicability. Within the framework of this paper, I have quite consciously devoted the least amount of space to the therapeutic side of Tibetan medicine. Tibetan medicine is not only of great theoretical interest, but it could also be practiced in the West. At the beginning I pointed out that the theoretical principles, the regligious background, indeed the whole system of Tibetan medicine have to be studied very carefully. In the West interest in Tibetan medicine is particularly great, and for exactly this reason in an age like ours which is only too willing to try out Oriental practices and miracle drugs, we need to guard ourselves against adopting uncritically detached fragments of the Tibetan medical system—meaningful in itself—and against a too hasty posing of questions concerning its applicability. Tibetan medicine is not some sort of technique which can be learned in a crash course. All Tibetan methods of treatment can only be applied successfully once the theoretical principles have been studied extensively and Tibetan doctors have supplied a through explanation of how these methods are to be put into practice.

Tibetan herbal therapy must be regarded with particular caution and a great deal of suspicion—there are considerable problems associated with this method of treatment. In many countries there will also be problems with the importing, production and application of the subtle Tibetan herbal preparations because of new pharmaceutical laws which require proof of the therapeutic effectiveness and the innocuousness of all pharmaceutics.

That is why we are fortunate in having certain typically Tibetan methods of treatment, moxibustion (cauterization) and blood-letting, which make us independent of the still-questionable herbal therapy. Thus these two Tibetan methods with their similarity to the Chinese ones are those we can apply first, once the constitutional type and the various indications have been recognized.

My altogether cautious, critical and reserved attitude regarding the applicability of Tibetan medicine in the West and my warning against a too hasty adoption of Tibetan methods of treatment are evident and I hope that I have made it clear in this short paper that superfluous philosophical speculations and premature, ill-considered and uncritical application of these methods of treatment would only place Tibetan medicine in danger of being written off as just another form of alternative medicine. We must ensure this does not happen. Tibetan medicine with all its precious, fascinating and valuable insights deserves much more than that—it must be preserved and carefully examined and studied.

NOTES

1. *rGyud bzhi* (*Four Treatises*) is the abbreviated title; the full title is *bDud rtsi snying po yan lag brgyad pa gsang ba man ngag gi rgyud* (*Secret Treatise of Instructions on the Eight-Branched Essence of Immortality*).
2. Martin Brauen has pointed out in his book *Impressionen aus Tibet* that Tibetan popular belief has never been properly considered, or at best, badly neglected, with the result that a one-sided picture of Tibet's religious heritage is often presented. I share his view—Tibetan medicine would be deprived of its colorful character if one were to leave out this important aspect.
3. M. Porkert, *Lehrbuch der chinesischen Diagnostik*, p. 13.
4. Elisabeth Finckh, *Foundations of Tibetan Medicine*, Vol. I. Watkins Publishing, London, 1978.

This paper was first published in *Tibetan Studies in Honour of Hugh Richardson*, Proceedings of the International Seminar on Tibetan Studies, Oxford 1979.

The System of Tibetan Medicine

According to the *rGyud bźi*

INTRODUCTION

The first step in researching into Tibetan medicine undoubtedly has to be the compilation of the medical terminology from the sources available. The standard work of the Tibetan doctors is the book *Four Treatises* or *Four Tantras* = *rGyud bźi* (abbreviated title). Thanks to the assistance of Tibetan doctors and Tibetologists, it has been possible to translate several important chapters of this book. Thus, a start has been made in the work of compiling a medical terminology from these texts.

The *Four Treatises* is a book made up of four parts. In part I the system of Tibetan medicine is described—symbolically—as a tree with 3 roots, 9 trunks, 47 branches and 224 leaves. The intention of this paper is to present in summarised form a description of the system; all the terms taken from the texts (283 of them) are given together with the equivalent Tibetan terms.

By the end of this paper, we trust that the immense practical significance of the Tibetan system will be apparent.

The 3 roots are described in part I of the *Four Treatises*:
Root A-Chapter 3
Root B-Chapter 4
Root C-Chapter 5.

THE TEXT

ROOT A

Arrangement (of the parts of the body and) bases of diseases = gnas lugs nad gźi

rGyud bźi, part 1, Chapter 3, fol. 6b, 7a, 7b, 8a of my block-print.

I, 1 srog ẖǰin gyen rgyu khyab byed me thur sel//
ẖju byed mdaṅs sgyur sgrub(7bl)mthoṅ mdog gsal lṅa//
rten myag myoṅ ćhim ẖbyor byed bco lṅaho//
2 daṅs ma khrag śa ćhil rus rkaṅ khu ba//
3 lus zuṅs bdun yin dri ma bśaṅ gci rṅul//
nad ni skyed par byed paẖi rgyu gsum ste//
de la lhan cig bskyed paẖi rkyen bźi yis//
ẖjug sgo rnam pa drug tu (7b3) źugs nas ni//
lus kyi stod smad bar du gnas bcas śiṅ//
rgyu bar byed paẖi lam ni bco lṅa ru//
na so yul dus dgu ru ẖphel byed de//
ẖbras bu srog gcod pa yi nad dgur smin//
ldog paẖi rgyu ni bcu daṅ gñis su ẖgyur//
(7b4) mdo don dril bas ćha graṅ gñis su ẖdus//

II,1 de la ẖdod chags źe sdaṅ gti mug gsum//
rluṅ mkhris bad kan rim pas skyed paẖi rgyu//
2 de la dus gdon zas daṅ spyod lam bźis//
de dag (7b5) ẖphel daṅ zad par gyur nas ni//
3 pags la gram źiṅ śa la rgyas pa daṅ//
rća ru rgyu źiṅ rus la źen pa daṅ//
don la ẖbab ciṅ snod du lhuṅ bar ẖgyur//
4 bad kan klad pa la brten stod na gnas//
mkhris pa mchin dri la brten bar na (7b6) gnas//

rluṅ ni dpyi rked la brten smad na gnas//
5 rus pa rna ba reg bya sñiṅ srog loṅ//
khrag rṅul mig daṅ mchin mkhris rgyu ma daṅ//
dvaṅs ma śa ćhil rkaṅ khu bśaṅ gci daṅ//
sna lce glo mcher pho mkhal lgaṅ pa rnams//
lus (8al) zuṅs dri ma dbaṅ po don snod lṅa//
rluṅ mkhris bad kan rgyu baẖi lam du bśad//
6 rgas pa rluṅ mi dar ma mkhris paẖi mi//
byis pa bad kan mi yin na sos gñan//
ṅad can graṅ ba rluṅ gi yul yin te//
(8a2) skam sa ćha gduṅ che ba mkhris paẖi yul//
rlan can snum pa bad kan yul du bśad//
rluṅ nad dbyar dus dgoṅs daṅ tho raṅs ldaṅ//
mkhris pa ston dus ñin dguṅ mćhan dguṅ ldaṅ//
bad kan dpyid dus srod daṅ sṅa (8a3) dro ldaṅ//
7 ẖćho ba gsum zad ẖdu ba gśed du babs//
sbyor ba mćhuṅs daṅ gnad du babs pa daṅ//
dus ẖdas rluṅ nad srog rten chad pa daṅ//
ćha ba la ẖdas graṅ ba gtiṅ ẖkhar ba//
zuṅs kyis mi thub rnam par ẖćhe ba (8a4) rnams//
ẖbras bu srog gcod nad dgu źes su bśad//
8 rluṅ mkhris bad kan źi daṅ ma źi ba//
gñis gñis bźi ru ldog pas bcu gñis so//
9 rluṅ daṅ bad kan graṅ ba chu yin te//
khrag daṅ mkhris pa ćha ba me ru ẖdod//

ROOT A — 2 trunks

Arrangement (of the parts of the body and) bases of disease
gnas lugs nad gźi

Trunk I — 3 branches

Not changed-*rnam par ma gyur pa*
i.e. Healthy organism

Branch 1 — 15 leaves

(Bases of) diseases-*nad*

Wind-*rluṅ*:

Sustaining life-*srog hjin*, moving upwards-*gyen rgyu*, penetrating-*khyab byed*, (accompanying) fire-*me*, removing downwards-*thur sel*

Bile-*mkhris pa*:

Causing digestion-*hju byed*, producing brightness (of chyle)-*mdaṅs sgyur*, satisfying (desires)-*sgrub*, causing vision-*mthoṅ byed*, making clear the color (of the skin)-*mdog gsal*

Phlegm-*bad kan*:

Supporting-*rten byed*, decomposing-*myag byed*, causing taste-*myoṅ byed*, causing satisfaction-*ĉhim byed*, causing to bind-*ẖbyor byed*

Branch 2 — 7 leaves

Constituents (of the body)-*lus zuṅs*

Chyle-*daṅs ma*, blood-*khrag*, flesh-*śa*, fat-*ĉhil*, bones-*rus pa*, marrow-*rkaṅ*, semen-*khu ba*

Branch 3 — 3 leaves

Impurities-*dri ma*

Faeces-*bśaṅ*, urine-*gcin*, sweat-*rṅul*

25 leaves

From trunk I also issue:

2 flowers=health and long life

3 fruits=religion, prosperity and happiness.

Trunk II — 9 branches

Changed-*rnam par gyur pa*

i.e. diseased organism

Branch 1 — 3 leaves

Producing (primary) causes-*rgyu*

Passion-*ẖdod chags* (wind), hate-*źe sdaṅ* (bile), delusion-*gti mug* (phlegm)

Branch 2 — 4 leaves

Promoting (secondary) causes-*rkyen*

Time-*dus*, demons-*gdon*, nutrition-*zas*, behavior-*spyod*

Branch 3 — 6 leaves

Means of entrance-*ẖjug sgo*

Skin-*pags pa*, flesh-*śa*, veins, nerves-*rća*, bones-*rus pa*, 5 solid organs=heart-*sñiṅ*, liver-*mchin pa*, lungs-*glo ba*, spleen-*mcher pa*, kidneys-*mkhal ma* (=*don*).

6 hollow organs=large intestine-*loṅ ka*, gall-*bladder-mkhris pa*, small intestine-*rgyu ma*, stomach-*pho ba*, urinary bladder-*lgaṅ pa, bsam seẖu (=snod).*

Branch 4 — 3 leaves

Places of residence (site)-*gnas*

Upper site-*stod na gnas* (phlegm), middle site-*bar na gnas* (bile), lower site-*smad na gnas* (wind)

Branch 5 — 15 leaves

Paths of circulation-*lam*

Combination of wind, bile and phlegm with:

1. Constituents of the body,
2. Impurities,
3. Sensory organs-*dbaṅ po*=ear-*rna ba*, touch-*reg bya*, eye-*mig*, nose-*sna*, tongue-*lce*
4. Hollow organs,
5. Solid organs

	Wind	Bile	Phlegm
Constituents of the body	1 Bones	6 Blood	11 Chyle, flesh, fat, marrow, semen
Impurities	2 [reg bya] "skin"	7 Sweat	12 Faeces, urine
Sensory organs	3 Ear [touch]	8 Eye	13 Nose, tongue
Solid organs (don)	4 Heart, [life-(-veins)]	9 Liver	14 Spleen, kidneys, lungs
Hollow organs (snod)	5 Large intestine	10 Gall bladder, small intestine	15 Stomach, urinary-bladder

Branch 6 9 leaves

1. Age-*na so*

   Old person-*rgas pa* (wind), young person-*mi dar ma* (bile), child-*byis pa* (phlegm)

2. Place-*yul*

   Fragrant-windy-*ṅad can*, cold-*graṅ ba* (wind diseases increase)

   Dry-*skam pa*, hot-*ĉha ba* (bile diseases increase)

   Damp-*rlan can*, oily-*snum pa* (phlegm diseases increase)

3. Time-*dus*

   Summer (rainy season)-*dbyar ka*, early evening-*dgoṅ*, at dawn-*tho raṅs* (wind diseases break out)

   Autumn-*ston ka*, noon-*ñin duṅ*, midnight-*mĉhan dguṅ* (bile diseases break out)

   Spring-*dpyid ka*, at dusk-*srod*, morning-*sṅa dro* (phlegm diseases break out)

Branch 7 9 leaves

Fruit (result)-*ẖbras bu*

1. Three lives have been completed-*ẖĉho ba gsum zad pa*
2. The conjunction has fallen into the (hands) of the executioner-*ẖdu ba gśed du babs pa*
3. Similar mixtures (of medicine)-*sbyor ba mĉhuṅs pa*
4. A vital spot is attacked (by weapons)-*gnad du babs pa*
5. The sustenance of life is cut off, (because) the time for the (treatment) of wind disease is over-*dus ẖdas rluṅ nad srog rten chad pa*
6. (The moment) (for treating a disease of) heat has been missed-*ĉha ba la ẖdas pa*
7. To be overcome by intense cold-*graṅ ba gtiṅ ẖkhar ba*
8. The constituents (of the body) are unable to tolerate (medical treatment)-*zuṅs kyis mi thub*
9. Severe persecution (by demons)-*rnam par ẖĉhe ba rnams*

Branch 8 12 leaves

Causes opposing (each other)-ldog rgyu

1 + + Wind-Bile	− − Wind-Bile	− + Wind-Bile	+ − Wind-Bile
+ + Wind-Phlegm	− − Wind-Phlegm	− + Wind-Phlegm	+ − Wind-Phlegm
+ + Bile-Phlegm	− − Bile-Phlegm	− + Bile-Phlegm	12 + − Bile-Phlegm

Through the progress of "reversible change" the diseases can be transformed from one component to another.

Branch 9 — 2 leaves

Principles-*mdo don*

Cold-*graṅ ba*

Heat-*ćha ba*

All diseases can be traced back to cold and heat.

63 leaves

Trunk I	3 branches	25 leaves
Trunk II	9 branches	63 leaves
Root A		88 leaves

THE TEXT

ROOT B

diagnosis=*ṅos ḫjin rtags*

rGyud bźi, part 1, Chapter 4, fol. 8a, 8b, 9a of my block-print

III,1 rluṅ gi lce ni dmar źiṅ skam la rćub//
mkhris lce bad kan skya sar mthug pos g-yogs//
bad kan skya gleg mdaṅs med ḫjam la rlon//
2 rluṅ gi chu ni chu ḫdra lbu ba che//
mkhris chu dmar ser rlaṅs che dri ma (8b3) dugs//
bad kan chu ni dkar la dri rlaṅs chuṅ//
IV,1 rluṅ gi rća ni rkyal stoṅ skabs su sdod//

2 mkhris paẖi rća ni mgyogs rgyas grims par ẖphar//
3 bad kan rća ni byiṅ rgud dal baẖo//
V,1 dri ba yaṅ la rćub paẖi zas spyod kyi//
2 (8b4) rkyen gyis g-yal ẖdar bya rmyaṅ graṅ śum byed//
dpyi daṅ rked pa rus ćhigs ma lus na//
gzer ba ṅes med ẖpho źiṅ stoṅ skyugs byed//
dbaṅ po mi gsal śes pa ẖćhub pa daṅ//
3 bkres dus na źiṅ *snum* bcud phan par ṅes//
rno źiṅ ćha (8b5) baẖi zas daṅ spyod lam gyis//
kha kha mgo na śa drod ćha ba daṅ//
3 stod gzer źu rjes na źiṅ *bsil* ba phan//
lci la snum paẖi zas daṅ spyod lam gyis//
daṅ ga mi bde kha zas ẖju ba dkaẖ//
skyug ciṅ kha mṅal pho ba ćhiṅ ste sgreg//
(8b6) lus sems lci la phyi naṅ gñis ka graṅ//
3 zos rjes mi bde zas spyod *dro* na ẖphrod//

ROOT B — 3 trunks

Diagnosis—ṅos hǰin rtags

Trunk III — 2 branches

Observation-*blta*

Branch 1 — 3 leaves

Tongue-*lce*

Red-dmar po, dry-*skam pa*, rough-*rćub pa* (wind)

Covered with thick, tawny phlegm-*bad kan skya sar mthug pos g-yogs* (bile)

Grey-*skya bo*, thick-*gleg*, lustreless-*mdaṅs med*, smooth-*hjam pa*, moist-*rlon pa* (phlegm)

Branch 2 — 3 leaves

Urine-*chu*

Like water-*chu ẖdra*, big bubbles-*lbu ba che* (wind)

Reddish-yellow-*dmar ser*, much vapor-*rlaṅs che*, hot smell-*dri ma dugs* (bile)

White-*dkar ba*, little odor-*dri chuṅ*, little vapor-*rlaṅs chuṅ* (phlegm).

6 leaves

Trunk IV 3 branches

Feeling (the pulse of the vein)-*reg pa*

Palpation

Branch 1 1 leaf

Swim-*rkyal*, empty-*stoṅ*, stopping at times-*skabs su sdod* (wind)

Branch 2 1 leaf

Beats quickly, spreads (and beats) subtly-*mgyogs rgyas grims par h̠phar* (bile)

Branch 3 1 leaf

Sink-*byiṅ*, weak-*rgud*, slow-*dal ba* (phlegm)

3 leaves

Trunk V 3 branches

Questioning-*dri ba*

Branch 1 3 leaves

Productive causes-*sloṅ rkyen*

Light-*yaṅ ba*, rough-*rćub pa* (wind)

Sharp-*rno ba*, hot-*ćha ba* (bile)

Heavy-*lci ba*, oily-*snum pa* (phlegm)

Branch 2 23 leaves

Conditions of illness-*na lugs*

Gaping, shuddering-*g-yal h̠dar*, stretching-*bya rmyaṅ*, shivering with cold-*graṅ śum byed*, pain in all bone-joints of the thigh and hip-*dpyi daṅ rked pa rus ćhigs ma lus na*, indefinite aches that change-*gzer ba ṅes med h̠pho*, making vomit (on an) empty (stomach)-*stoṅ skyugs byed*, the sense-organs are not bright-*dbaṅ po mi gsal*, knowledge is stifled-*śes pa h̠ćhub pa*, pains at the time of hunger-*bkres dus na* (wind=9)

Bitter taste-*kha kha*, headaches-*mgo na*, hot flesh (fever)-*śa drod ćha ba*, aches in the upper part (of the body)-*stod gzer*, pains after digestion-*źu rjes na* (bile=5)

Uncomfortable appetite-*daṅ ga mi bde*, difficulty in digesting food-*kha zas h̠ju ba dkah̠*, vomiting-*skyug*, (bad taste in) the hollow of the mouth-*kha mṅal*, distended stomach-*pho ba ćhiṅ*, eructation-*sgreg*, body and mind being heavy (together)-

lus sems lci, being cold both outside and inside-*phyi naṅ gñis ka graṅ*, discomfort after eating-*zos rjes mi bde.* (phlegm=9)

Branch 3 — 3 leaves

(Habits in connection with) food-*zas*

Oily-*snum pa* (wind)
Cool-*bsil ba* (bile)
Warm-*dro ba* (phlegm)

		29 leaves
Trunk III	2 branches	6 leaves
Trunk IV	3 branches	3 leaves
Trunk V	3 branches	29 leaves
Root B		38 leaves

THE TEXT

ROOT C

Therapy=*gso thabs*

rGyud bźi, part 1, Chapter 5, fol. 9a, 9b of my block-print

VI,1 rta boṅ ẖphyi ba lo śa śa chen daṅ//
hbru mar lo mar bu ram sgog skya bćoṅ//
2 ẖo ma lca ba ra mñe zan chaṅ daṅ//
bur chaṅ rus chaṅ rluṅ nad can gyi (9a3) zas//
3 ba raẖi źo dar mar gsar ri dvags śa//
ra śa skom śa gsar pa chag ćhe daṅ//
4 skyabs daṅ khur ćhod chab ćha chu bsil daṅ//
bskol graṅs mkhris paẖi nad kyi zas su bśad//
5 lug daṅ g-yag rgod gcan gzan ña yi śa//
(9a4) sbraṅ rći skam saẖi ẖbru rñiṅ zan dron daṅ//
6 ẖbri yi źo dar gar chaṅ chu skol ni//
bad kan nad ǵzi can gyis bsten par bya//
VII,1 rluṅ la dro sar yid ẖoṅ grogs bsten źiṅ//
2 mkhris paẖi nad la bsil sar dal bar bsdad//
3 bad (9a5) kan nad la rćol bcag dro sa bsten//
IIX,1,2 rluṅ la mṅar skyur lan ćha snum lci ẖjam//
3,4 mṅar kha bska bsil sla rtul mkhris paẖi sman//

5,6 ćha skyur bska rno rćub yaṅ bad kan no//
ro nus de la sbyor ba źi sbyaṅ gñis//
źi byed rluṅ la khu ba (9a6) sman mar gñis//
mkhris paẖi nad la thaṅ daṅ cur nis bsten//
bad kan nad la ril bu tres sam sbyar//
7 khu ba rus khu bcud bźi mgo khrol te//
8 sman mar jā ti sgog skya ẖbras bu gsum//
rća ba lṅa daṅ sman chen dag la (9bl) sbyar//
9 ma nu sle tres tig ta ẖbras buẖi thaṅ//
10 ga bur can dan gur gum cu gaṅ phye//
11 bćan dug ćhva sna rnams kyi ril bu daṅ//
12 tres sam se ẖbru da lis rgod ma kha//
ćhva daṅ coṅ źi bsregs paẖi thal sman no//
sbyoṅ byed (9b2) rluṅ gi nad la ẖjam rći ste//
mkhris pa bśal la bad kan skyugs kyis sbyaṅ//
13 ẖjam rći sle ẖjam bkru ẖjam bkru ma slen//
14 bśal la spyi bśal sgos bśal drag daṅ ẖjam//
15 skyugs la drag skyugs ẖjam (9b3) skyugs gñis su sbyar//
IX, 1 dpyad du bsku mñe hor gyi me bćaẖ daṅ//
2 rṅul dbyuṅ gtar ga chu yi ẖphrul ẖkhor daṅ//
3 dugs daṅ me bćaẖ rim bźin dpyad kyis bcos//

ROOT C 4 trunks
Therapy—gso thabs

Trunk VI 6 branches
Nutrition-*zas*
Branch 1 10 leaves
food-*zas*

Horse (flesh)-rta, donkey (flesh)-*boṅ*, marmot (flesh)-*ẖphyi ba*, flesh that is a year old-*lo śa*, human flesh-*śa chen*, sesame oil-*ẖbru mar*, oil that is a year old-*lo mar*, crude sugar-*bu ram*, garlic-*sgog skya*, onions-*bćoṅ*, (wind)

Branch 2 4 leaves
drink-*skom*

Milk-*ẖo ma*, carrot and onion soup-*lca ba ra mñe zan chaṅ*, liquid (extract of) crude sugar-*bur chaṅ*, bone soup-*rus chaṅ* (wind)

Branch 3 — 9 leaves

food-*zas*

Curds of cow and goat-*ba ra*h̲*i źo*, buttermilk-*dar*, fresh butter-*mar gsar*, game flesh-*ri dvags śa*, goat flesh-*ra śa*, fresh flesh of animals of mixed breed-*skom śa gsar pa*, young barley-*chag ćhe*, "skyabs" herbs-*skyabs*,[1] dandelions-*khur ćhod* (bile)

Branch 4 — 3 leaves

drink-*skom*

hot water-*chab ćha*, cool water-*chu bsil, boiled and cooled water-chu bskol graṅs* (bile)

Branch 5 — 6 leaves

food-*zas*

Sheep (flesh)-*lug*, wild yak-*g-yag rgod*, beasts of prey-*gcan gzan*, fish flesh-*ña yi śa*, honey-*sbraṅ rći*, hot pap of old grain from dry land-*skam sa*h̲*i* h̲*bru rñiṅ zan dron* (phlegm)

Branch 6 — 3 leaves

drink-*skom*

Curds and buttermilk of the yak-h̲*bri yi źo dar*, strong beer-*gar chaṅ*, boiled water-*chu skol* (phlegm)

35 leaves

Trunk VII — 3 branches

Behavior-*spyod*

Branch 1 — 2 leaves

Keep agreeable company-*yid* h̲*oṅ grogs bsten*,
Warm place-*dro sa* (wind)

Branch 2 — 2 leaves

Sit calmly-*dal bar bsdad*,
Cool place-*bsil sa* (bile)

Branch 3 — 2 leaves

Walk energetically-*rćol bcag*
Warm place-*dro sa* (phlegm)

6 leaves

Trunk IIX 15 branches

Medicaments-*sman*

Branch 1 3 leaves

Taste-*ro*

Sweet-*mṅar ba*, sour-*skyur ba*, saline-*lan ćhva ba* (wind)

Branch 2 3 leaves

Potency-*nus pa*

Oily-*snum pa*, heavy-*lci ba*, smooth-*ḫjam pa* (wind)

Branch 3 3 leaves

Taste-*ro*

Sweet-*mṅar ba*, bitter-*kha ba*, astringent-*bska ba* (bile)

Branch 4 3 leaves

Potency-*nus pa*

Cool-*bsil ba*, thin-*sla ba, blunt-rtul ba* (bile)

Branch 5 3 leaves

Taste-*ro*

Pungent-*ćha ba*, sour-*skyur ba*, astringent-*bska ba* (phlegm)

Branch 6 3 leaves

Potency-*nus pa*

Sharp-*rno ba*, rough-*rćub pa*, light-*yaṅ ba* (phlegm)

Branch 7 3 leaves

Soups-*khu ba* (making calm)

Soup from bones-*rus khu*, the four juices-*bcud bźi, "mgo khrol"-mgo khrol*[2], (wind).

Branch 8 5 leaves

Medicinal oils-*sman mar* (making calm)

Nard-*jā ti*, garlic-*sgog skya*, the three fruits-*ḫbras bu gsum*[3], the five roots-*rća ba lṅa*, aconites-*sman chen* (wind)

Branch 9 4 leaves

Syrups-*thaṅ* (making calm)

Orrisroot-*ma nu*, guduch-*sle tres*, chirata-*tig ta*, the three fruits-*ḫbras bu gsum* (bile)

Branch 10 4 leaves

Powders-*cur ni* (making calm)

Camphor-*ga bur*, sandal-*ćan dan*, saffron-*gur gum*, bamboo manna-*cu gaṅ* (bile)

Branch 11 2 leaves

Pills-*ril bu* (making calm)

Aconite-*bĉan dug*, varioius kinds of salt-*ĉhva sna rnams* (phlegm)

Branch 12 5 leaves

Pastes-*tres sam* (making calm)

Pomegranates-*se ḫbru*, rhododendrons-*da li*, "mare face"-*rgod ma kha*, alkaline medicaments (made) from burnt salt-*ĉhva bsregs paḫi thal sman*, white stone-*coṅ źi* (phlegm)

Branch 13 3 leaves

Oily enemas-*ḫjam rĉi* (making clean)

Mild-*sle ḫjam*, purgative-*bkru ḫjam*, purgative-not mild-*bkru ma slen* (wind)

Branch 14 4 leaves

Laxatives-*bśal sman* (making clean)

General-*spyi*, particular-*sgos*, severe-*drag*, mild-*ḫjam*

Branch 15 2 leaves

Emetics-*skyugs sman* (making clean)

Severe-*drag*, mild-*ḫjam* (phlegm)

50 leaves

Trunk IX 3 branches

Treatments (external)-*dpyad*

Branch 1 2 leaves

Inunction with massage-*bsku mñe*, Mongolian (type) cauterization-*hor gyi me bĉaḫ* (wind)

Branch 2 3 leaves

Production of sweat-*rṅul dbyuṅ*, bloodletting-*gtar ga*, the magic water-wheel-*chu yi ḫphrul ḫkhor* (bile)

Branch 3 2 leaves

Heat treatments-*dugs*, cauterization-*me bćah̲* (phlegm) 7 leaves

Trunk VI	6 branches	35 leaves
Trunk VII	3 branches	6 leaves
Trunk IIX	15 branches	50 leaves
Trunk IX	3 branches	7 leaves
Root C		98 leaves

Root A	88 leaves
Root B	38 leaves
Root C	98 leaves
	224 leaves

SUMMARY

Although Tibetan medicine has been greatly influenced by Indian and Chinese medicine, it has, however, most definitely developed a distinctive character of its own. The System described in this paper is without doubt of Tibetan origin.

The System enables us to determine the following:

1. It is possible to compile a medical terminology.
2. The three-part division which is typical of Tibetan medicine is unmistakable.
3. The nine disciplines of Tibetan medicine are described—together with their inter-relations.
4. A systematic description of Tibetan medicine is possible if we follow the System outlined in the *Four Treatises*.
5. As far as practice of Tibetan medicine is concerned, the texts show that the three types: wind, bile and phlegm are recognized by means of diagnosis; specific methods of treatment and medicines are assigned to the three types.

The System

			Trunk IX Treatments 3 branches 7 leaves
		Trunk V Questioning 3 branches 29 leaves	*Trunk IIX* Medicines 15 branches 50 leaves
	Trunk II Diseased organism 9 branches 63 leaves	*Trunk IV* Palpation 3 branches 3 leaves	*Trunk VII* Behavior 3 branches 6 leaves
	Trunk I Healthy organism 3 branches 25 leaves	*Trunk III* Observation 2 branches 6 leaves	*Trunk VI* Nutrition 6 branches 35 leaves
3 9 47 224	Root A *Arrangement* 2 Trunks 12 Branches 88 Leaves	Root B *Diagnosis* 3 Trunks 8 Branches 38 Leaves	Root C *Therapy* 4 Trunks 27 Branches 98 Leaves

NOTES

1. *skyabs.*
   According to the doctors at Dharamsala: a sort of dandelion (communicated in writing)
2. *mgo khrol.*
   According to the doctors at Dharamsala: old and ground sheep's head shoup (communicated in writing)
3. *ḫbras bu gsum*, the three fruits: the three myrobalans
   ā ru ra chebulic myrobalan (Terminalia Chebula)
   ba ru ra beleric myrobalan (Terminalia Bellerica)
   skyu ru ra emblic myrobalan (Phyllanthus Emblica)

This article is a short summary of *Foundations of Tibetan Medicine*, Vol. I, 1978 and *Foundations of Tibetan Medicine*, Vol. II, 1985, Robinson Books, London WC2H OLU.

Notes on Pulsology

INTRODUCTION

Before making use of Tibetan therapeutic methods, it is important to study their diagnostic methods and also to point out the difficulties.

Tibetan medicine has three diagnostic methods: Observation (*blta*), Palpation=pulse diagnosis (*reg pa*) and Questioning (*dri ba*). Pulse diagnosis is seen as the most important method of diagnosis because of the information obtained in this way about the functions of the organs. We want to start with some theoretical foundations derived from the texts. Pulse diagnosis is described in the Tibetan standard work, the book *rGyud bźi*[1]—Four Treatises (T), (part 4, chapter 1) and in the *Vaiḍūrya sṅon po*[2] (V)(part4, chapter1), the famous commentary on the *rGyud bźi* of Sde srid saṅs rgyas rgya mćho. Pulse diagnosis belongs to the Root B of the System of Tibetan medicine (3 branches, 3 leaves).

The first step is the connection between the three "humors"— wind, bile and phlegm—and the pulses:

1T4, 7b
rluṅ gi rća ni rkyal stoṅ skabs su sdod m̀khris paẖi
rća ni mgyogs rgyas grims par ẖphar/bad kan rća ni
byiṅ rgud dal baẖo//

"The pulse of (a person suffering from) wind (disease) swims, is empty and stops at times. The pulse of (a person suffering from) bile (disease), beats quickly, spreads (and beats) subtly. The pulse of (a person suffering from) phlegm (disease) sinks (to the bottom) and is weak and slow."

Continuing with another text of the rGyud bźi:

1T3, 7b

rus pa rna ba reg bya sñiṅ srog loṅ/khrag rṅul mig
daṅ mchin mkhris rgyu ma daṅ/dvaṅs ma śa ćhil rkaṅ
khu bśaṅ gci daṅ/sna lce glo mcher pho mkhal lgaṅ
pa rnams/lus zuṅs dri ma dbaṅ po don snod lṅa/rluṅ
mkhris bad kan rgyu baẖi lam du bśad//

"Bones, ears, touch, heart, life (-veins) and large intestine; blood, sweat, eyes, liver, gallbladder and small intestine; and chyle, flesh, fat, marrow, semen, faeces, urine, nose, tongue, lungs, spleen, stomach, kidneys and urinary bladder; (each of the) five (categories)—constituents of the body, impurities, sensory organs, solid organs and hollow organs—is said to be a path of circulation of wind, bile and phlegm."

Conclusion

The classification of organs into groups is noteworthy[3]

(1) The solid organs=*don*

1. heart-*sñiṅ*, 2. liver-*mchin pa*, 3. lungs-*glo ba*, 4. spleen-*mcher pa*, 5. kidneys-*mkhal ma*.

(2) The hollow organs=*snod*

1. large intestine-*loṅ ka*, 2. gallbladder-*mkhris pa*, 3. small intestine-*rgyu ma*, 4. stomach-*pho ba*, 5. urinary bladder-*lgaṅ pa* (6. *bsam seẖu*)[4].

It is a fact that these groups of organs are considered the "starting-point" of Tibetan pulses. We now have to consider why these groups are of such importance in understanding Tibetan pulse diagnosis.

CLASSIFICATION

Pulse diagnosis is divided into 13 sections.

4T1,2b

sṅon ẖgro zas spyod bslab daṅ blta dus bstan/blta gnas mnan ćhad blta ćhul śes pa yis /tha mal rća la rća rgyud gsum du brtag/dus bźiẖi rća la khams lṅa ẖbyuṅ ba rći / ṅo mćhar rća bdun nad med mi la blta/nad daṅ nad med ẖphar baẖi graṅs las dpags/spyi daṅ bye brag rća yis nad ṅos bzuṅ/ ẖchi rća gsum gyis ẖćho ẖchi kha dmar gdags/gdon rća glo bur ye ẖbrog rim gro ẖbogs/ćhe rtags bla yi rća la brtag pa ste/spyi don bcu gsum reg paẖi mdor bstan yin//

THE 13 SECTIONS:

I. Preceding food and behavior (*sṅon ẖgro zas spyod bslab*)
II. Time (*dus*)
III. Place (*gnas*)
IV. Amount of pressure (*mnan ćhad*)
V. Way, manner (to examine the pulse) (*ćhul*)
VI. Character of the three pulses (*rća rgyud gsum*)
VII. Pulses of the four seasons (*dus bźiẖi rća*)
IIX. The seven wonder (divination) pulses (*ṅo mćhar rća bdun*)
IX. Healthy and diseased (pulses) (*nad daṅ nad med*)
X. General and specific pulses (*spyi daṅ bye brag rća*)
XI. Three death pulses (*ẖchi rća gsum*)
XII. Demon (spirit) pulses (*gdon rća*)
XIII. Superior pulse (*bla yi rća*)

This paper deals with the first five points.

4V1,17a

I. Preceding food and behavior *(sṅon ẖgro zas spyod bslab)*

It is important that wind, bile and phlegm are in a good equilibrium. Therefore the patient is not allowed to have alcoholic drinks and heavy food during the evening before the pulse diagnosis. The patient should be relaxed. The doctor—for his part—should be in a good mental and physical condition.

4V1,17a

II. Time *(dus)*

The best time to examine the pulse is the early morning. The patient should have an empty stomach or, at least, not have eaten or drunk much.

4V1,17b

III. Place *(gnas)*

Tibetan doctors distinguish three positions at which the pulse can be felt: the upper pulses (head), the middle pulses (hand) and the lower pulses (foot). The hand palpation is the one which is mostly practiced. The doctor uses his right hand to examine the pulses on the left-hand side of the patient and his left hand for the pulses on the right-hand side of the patient. The palpation is carried out with the index finger (*mĉhon*), the middle finger (*kan ma*) and the ring finger (*chag*). The fingers must be in a straight line and should not touch each other.

The doctor takes the patient's hand and bends it so that the furrows of the wrist can be easily seen. Then, the doctor takes the patient's other hand and places the distal thumb phalanx of this hand on the proximal furrow of the other hand.

Thus the first pulse position is indicated by the distance between the relevant thumb phalanx and the hand furrow of the patient. The doctor now places his three above-mentioned fingers on this spot.

4V1,19a

IV. Amount of pressure *(mnan ĉhad)*

The pressure exerted by each of the three fingers is different, with the index finger exerting the least pressure, to feel the skin; the middle finger to feel the flesh; and the ring finger to feel the bone.

4V1,19b

V. Way, manner *(ĉhul)*

With women it is the pulse of the right hand which is examined first, with men the pulse of the left hand. I have often seen Tibetan doctors explain the examination in a typical way; on the finger tips of his own palpating fingers[5] the doctor describes the positions which are to be palpated: two organs are assigned to his left and right finger tips (see anatomical tables).

The positions. First we repeat the "starting point": (1) The solid organs (*don*): heart, liver, lungs, spleen, kidneys and (2) The hollow organs (*snod*): large intestine, gallbladder, small intestine, stomach, urinary bladder, *bsam seḫu*. After that we will analyze the text.

> 4T1,3a
>
> mćhon gyi ḫog tu sñiṅ daṅ rgyu maḫi rća /kan gyi ḫog tu mcher pa pho baḫi rća/chag gi ḫog tu mkhal g-yon bsam se brtag/ćhon ḫog loṅ kan ḫog mchin mkhris rća/chag ḫog mkhal ma g-yas daṅ lgaṅ pa brtag//

"The pulses of heart and small intestine under the index finger. The pulses of spleen and stomach under the middle finger. (The pulses) of the left kidney and *bsam seḫu* are to be palpated under the ring finger. (left-hand patient)

The pulses of the lungs and the large intestine under the index finger. Under the middle finger liver and gallbladder. (The pulses) of the right kidney and the urinary bladder are to be palpated under the ring finger. (right-hand patient)"

Result: no reference to the positions of the organs with regard to the upper and lower divisions. Consequently, other sources must be consulted.

The *rGyud bźi* is translated into Chinese. The title is *Sibu yidian* (Yongnian Li, transl; Beijing 1983). The following passage is from p. 404.

> Shouxian bingren zuoshou yishi you, cunmai zhi xia xin yu xiaochang zhu, guanmai zhi xia pi yu weifu qiu,

chimai zhi xia zuoshen sanjiao zhen. Bingren youshou yishi zuoshou kan, cun xia fei yu dachang guan gandan, chi xia ke zhen youshen he pangguang.

"At first the right hand of the doctor (takes) the left hand of the patient. Under the index-finger-pulse heart and small intestine are palpated. Under the middle-finger-pulse spleen and stomach are palpated. Under the ring-finger-pulse left kidney and *sanjiao* are palpated.

"If the doctor's left hand (takes) the patient's right hand to palpate: under the index finger lungs and large intestine, (under) the middle finger liver and gallbladder, under the ring finger right kidney and urinary bladder can be palpated."

Result: no reference to the positions of the organs with regard to the upper and lower divisions.

The translation points out: (1) index finger=*cun* (tib. *mćhon*), middle finger=*guan* (tib. *kan ma*), ring finger=*chi* (tib. *chag*). (2) Translation of the term *bsam seẖu*=*sanjiao.*

Bai ḍū rya sṅon po (V̱aiḍūrya=Sanskrit)

4V1,19b

lag pa g-yon pa la sman paẖi lag pa g-yas pas brtag ste/ji ltar źe na ćhon gyi yar zur gyi ẖog sñiṅ daṅ/mar zur gyi ẖog tu rgyu maẖi rća me khams kyi yul daṅ/de bźin du kan gyi yar zur gyi ẖog tu mcher pa daṅ mar zur du pho baẖi rća saẖi khams kyi yul/chag gi yar zur gyi ẖog/tu mkhal ma g-yon daṅ mar zur gyi ẖog tu bsam seẖu chu khams rnams rim bźin brtag par byaẖo/blta bya nad paẖi lag pa g-yas pa la sman paẖi g-yon pas blta ste/ćhon ẖog gi yar zur du glo ba daṅ mar zur du loṅ lcags khams/kan ẖog gi yar zur du mchin pa daṅ mar zur du mkhris rća śiṅ khams/chag gi ẖog yar zur du mkhal ma g-yas daṅ/mar zur du lgaṅ paẖi rća chu khams rnams yin pa ltar//

Left hand of the patient:

(1) Under the upper (*yar*) side (edge, corner, division) (*zur*) of the index finger: the heart. Under the lower side (*mar zur*): the small intestine; region of the element fire (*me*).

(2) Under the upper side of the middle finger: the spleen. Under the lower side: the stomach; region of the element earth (*sa*).
(3) Under the upper side of the ring finger: the left kidney. Under the lower side: the *bsam seḫu*; region of the element water (*chu*).

Right hand of the patient:
(1) Under the upper side of the index finger: the lungs. Under the lower side: the large intestine; region of the element iron (*lcags*).
(2) Under the upper side of the middle finger: the liver. Under the lower side: the gallbladder; region of the element wood (*śiṅ*)
(3) Under the upper side of the ring finger: the right kidney. Under the lower side: the urinary bladder; region of the element water (*chu*).

Another source is
sman dpyad zla baḫi rgyal po
"Medical Investigation of Lunar King"[6]
(chapter 55;57,58)

> bud med g-yas la brtag par bya sman paḫi g-yon pas/
> g-yon paḫi ćhon la ya zur sñiṅ daṅ ma zur rgyu/kan
> la mchin daṅ mkhris pa ste/chag la mkhal g-yas lgaṅ
> phugs so(phug?) g-yas paḫi ćhon la glo daṅ loṅ/kan
> la mcher pa pho baḫi/chag la mkhal g-yon bsam seḫu//

"The right (hand) of the woman is palpated with the left (hand) of the doctor. Upper side (corner, division) (*ya zur*) of the left index finger: heart and lower side (*ma zur*): small intestine. Middle finger: liver and gallbladder. Ring finger: right kidney (and) urinary bladder.

"Right index finger: lungs and large intestine. Middle finger: spleen (and) stomach. Ring finger: left kidney (and) *bsam seḫu*."

Conclusion. The *don*=solid organs (heart, liver, lungs, spleen, kidneys) correspond to the upper sides (*yar zur*).

The *snod*=hollow organs (large intestine, gallbladder, small intestine, stomach, urinary bladder, *bsam seh̠u*) correspond to the lower sides (*mar zur*).

[The *don*=solid organs are palpated with the right side of the finger tip.

The *snod*=hollow organs are palpated with the left side of the finger tip (see Note 5).]

Tibetan pulses

left hand of the patient

positions	organ		division	finger tip
I	heart	don	upper	right side
index finger	small intestine	snod	lower	left side
II	spleen	don	upper	right side
middle finger	stomach	snod	lower	left side
III				
ring finger	left kidney	don	upper	right side
	bsam seh̠u	snod	lower	left side

Position I: female pulses are interchanged

right hand of the patient

I				
index finger	lungs	don	upper	right side
	large intestine	snod	lower	left side
II				
middle finger	liver	don	upper	right side
	gallbladder	snod	lower	left side
III				
ring finger	right kidney	don	upper	right side
	urinary bladder	snod	lower	left side

CHINESE PULSES

According to traditional Chinese medicine there are two main principles—yin and yang.

There are two groups of organs:

zang=yin=solid organs	*fu*=yang=hollow organs
1. lungs (*Fei*)	large intestine (*Da Chang*)
2. spleen (*Pi*)	stomach (*Wei*)
3. heart (*Xin*)	small intestine (*Xiao Chang*)
4. kidney (*Shen*)	urinary gladder (*Pang Guang*)
(5.) Xin Bao	San Jiao
6. liver (*Gan*)	gallbladder (*Dan*)

There are twelve so-called meridians; the "energy" (*Qi*) flows through these meridians in a certain invariable sequence: lungs—large intestine—stomach— spleen—heart—small intestine—urinary bladder—kidneys—*Xin Bao—San Jiao*—gallbladder—liver.

The table points out that the meridians are double-paired, for many reasons. The pulse at the radial artery of the wrist is divided into three zones; each has a lower and an upper position. The "starting-point" was: the solid organs=*don* (Tibetan)—*zang*=yin (Chinese) and the hollow organs=*snod* (Tibetan)—*fu*=yang (Chinese). The comparison pointed out the identity of these groups. The question is: can we find the same identity with regard to the pulse positions? The following comparison points out in what respects the Tibetan and the Chinese pulses agree and differ.

Positions

Position I. Distinction between male and female pulses; right and left hand interchanged.

Position II. The groups are reversed.

Position III. Tibetan pulses: kidneys are palpated on both hands. Left hand: *bsam sehu*. Chinese pulses: left side: kidneys and urinary bladder, right side: *Xin Bao, San Jiao.*

Chinese pulses

left hand of the patient

positions	organ		division	
I	heart	zang	lower	yin
index finger	small intestine	fu	upper	yang
II				
middle finger	liver	zang	lower	yin
	gallbladder	fu	upper	yang
III				
ring finger	kidneys	zang	lower	yin
	urinary bladder	fu	upper	yang

right hand of the patient

I				
index finger	lungs	zang	lower	yin
	large intestine	fu	upper	yang
II				
middle finger	spleen	zang	lower	yin
	stomach	fu	upper	yang
III				
ring finger	Xin Bao	zang	lower	yin
	San Jiao	fu	upper	yang

Method of feeling

Tibetan:

don=solid organs upper   *snod*=hollow organs lower

Chinese:

zang=solid organs lower   *fu*=hollow organs upper.

Conclusion:

All groups are interchanged according to upper and lower method of feeling. This comparison reveals a great difference—a most important distinction.

Comparison: Tibetan and Chinese pulses

Positions	Left hand patient	Right hand patient
I index finger woman don snod	*Tibetan* lungs *glo ba* large intestine *loṅ ka*	*Tibetan* heart *sñiṅ* small intestine *rgyu ma*
I index finger man don *snod*	heart *sñiṅ* small intestine *rgyu ma*	lungs *glo ba* large intestine *loṅ ka*
I index finger zang fu	*Chinese* heart small intestine	*Chinese* lungs large intestine
II middle finger don snod	*Tibetan* spleen *mcher pa* stomach *pho ba*	*Tibetan* liver *mchin pa* gallbladder *mkhris pa*
II middle finger zang fu	*Chinese* liver gallbladder	*Chinese* spleen stomach
III ring finger don snod	*Tibetan* left kidney *mkhal g-yon* *bsam seẖu*	*Tibetan* right kidney *mkhal g-yas* urinary bladder *lgaṅ pa*
III ring finger zang fu	*Chinese* kidneys urinary bladder	*Chinese* Xin Bao San Jiao

Tibetan Pulses

left hand patient	right hand patient					
heart	lungs	I	solid organ	don	upper	right
small intestine	large intestine	index finger	hollow organ	snod	lower	left
spleen	liver	II	solid organ	don	upper	right
stomach	gallbladder	middle finger	hollow orga	snod	lower	left
left kidney	right kidney	III	solid organ	don	upper	right
bsam seẖu	urinary bladder	ring finger	hollow organ	snod	lower	left

Chinese Pulses

left hand patient	right hand patient				
heart	lungs	I	solid organ	zang-yin	lower
small intestine	large intestine	index finger	hollow organ	fu-yang	upper
liver	spleen	II	solid organ	zang-yin	lower
gallbladder	stomach	middle finger	hollow organ	fu-yang	upper
kidneys	Xin Bao	III	solid organ	zang-yin	lower
urinary bladder	San Jiao	ring finger	hollow organ	fu-yang	upper

FINAL OBSERVATIONS

The fact that Tibetan doctors most probably adopted the pulse diagnosis for the most part from the Chinese is confirmed by the texts presented in this essay. To conclude this fifth section, three fundamental observations need to be made:

1. The solid organs, which in accordance with their yin character are situated on the inside, i.e. underneath, are palpated by the Tibetans on the outside, i.e. on the surface. Chinese pulse diagnosis teaches us just the opposite, as we have discovered. This fact is a source of extraordinary disquiet to any healer making use of acupuncture—and rightly so! However, it can be seen that Tibetan pulse diagnosis is more in line with the anatomical structure of the body in some respects than the Chinese one is. After all, it is more logical to palpate the gallbladder and liver, situated on the right-hand side of the body, with the right hand. Moreover, it also seems more logical to palpate the kidneys, situated on both sides of the body, with both hands.

2. This brings us to the next point. In this short essay we have merely been dealing with the present state of affairs in pulsology. But pulse diagnosis has undergone a lengthy development process in the course of its history stretching back over thousands of years. However, since this development cannot be described in this essay, we have added a table to illustrate this. As one can see from this, there were times when the kidneys, to take one example, were palpated on both hands. Pulse diagnosis has thus been subject to a process of constant change. Therefore, it is by no means out of the question that the typical Asiatic principle of change could continue to have its effect on pulse diagnosis. In other words, the present status need not be the ultimate stage of development.

3. Pulse diagnosis is extremely difficult to learn for us Western doctors because our sense organs are not as finely developed as those of the Asiatic healer. But, above all, there is the fact that pulse diagnosis is regarded as very dubious by Western medicine because it is difficult to objectify. However, there have

Pulse Position Correlations
Summary of Opinions from Major Authoritative Sources

Position		*Nei Jing* 1st cent. B.C.E.	*Nan Jing* c. 200 C.E.	Wang Shu-he's Classic of Pulse c. 280 C.E.	Li Shi-zhen's Pulse Studies 1564 C.E.	Zhang Jie-bing's Complete Book 1624 C.E.
Left Hand						
First	Deep	Heart	Arm *Shao-yin*	Heart	Heart	Heart
	Superficial	Sternum	Arm *Tai-yang*	Small Intestine		Pericardium
Second	Deep	Liver	Leg *Jue-yin*	Liver	Liver	Liver
	Superficial	Diaphragm	Leg *Shao-yang*	Gall Bladder		Gall Bladder
Third	Deep	Kidney	Leg *Shao-yin*	Kidney	Kidney	Kidney
	Superficial	Abdomen	Leg *Tai-yang*	Bladder	(Life Gate)	Bladder Large Intestine
Right Hand						
First	Deep	Lungs	Arm *Tai-yin*	Lungs	Lungs	Lungs
	Superficial	Chest	Arm *Yang-ming*	Large Intestine		Sternum
Second	Deep	Stomach	Leg *Tai-yin*	Spleen	Spleen	Spleen
	Superficial	Spleen	Leg *Yang-ming*	Stomach		Stomach
Third	Deep	Kidney	(text unclear)	Kidney (Life Gate)	Kidney (Life Gate)	Kidney
	Superficial	Abdomen		Triple Burner		Triple Burner Life Gate Small Intestine

In: Kaptchuk, T. J. "Chinese Medicine"; p. 300.

been tests which have objectified pulse diagnosis. For example, the French researcher Niboyet (1953) recorded the pulse using a sphygmograph, and Morita, a Japanese scientist, provided proof of the pulse through a pulsogram.

It is absolutely essential that further investigations are carried out to prove the reality of pulse diagnosis. When pulse diagnosis becomes more objectifiable, it would be possible to clear up the differences between Tibetan and Chinese pulsology described here.

NOTES

1. *rGyud bźi:* abbreviated title. Title of part 4 (67 folios) *bdud rći sñiṅ po yan lag brgyad pa gsaṅ ba man ṅag gi rgyud las dum bu bźi pa phyi maḫi rgyud*

   Blockprint in my possession; present from my teacher Dr. Yeshe Donden, Dharamsala 1962.
2. *Vaiḍūrya sṅon po:* abbreviated title. Title of part 4 (251 folios)

   gso ba rig paḫi bstan bcos sman blaḫi dgoṅs rgyan rgyud bźiḫi gsal byed bai ḍūr sṅon poḫi phreṅ ba las dum bu bźi pa phyi ma rgyud kyi rnam bśad

   Reproduction (Bai ḍūr sṅon po): Smanrtsis Shesrig Series, ed. T. Y. Tashigangpa, (Vols. 51-54), Leh 1973.
3. R. E. Emmerick "Sources of the *Rgyud-bźi*," *Zeitschrift der Morgenländischen Gesellschaft.* Suppl. III, 2, 1977; 1135,1136: "that the body organs are in Indian medical literature simply listed in various ways, whereas they are classified into five solid (Tibetan: *don lṅa*) and six hollow (Tibetan: *snod drug*) organs in the *Rgyud-bźi* in exact agreement with the Chinese system of classification of yin and yang organs." (1) See E. Finckh, "Grundlagen tibetischer Heilkunde," Vol. I, 1975; 74, 94. And "Foundations of Tibetan Medicine," Vol. I, 1978; 72. "This classification of organs into these groups is identical with the Chinese. The fact that the division of the organs into groups

described above is identical in Tibetan and Chinese medicine (*zang-yin-don; fu-yang-snod*) indicates that the Tibetans very probably adopted the pulse diagnosis form the Chinese."

4. *bsam seẖu*

Some explanations: (1) H. A. Jäschke, (A Tibetan-English Dictionary; 319): "...urinary bladder and spermatic vessels (in the female: uterus)..."

(2) In many Tibetan books the term *bsam seẖu* is translated: "reproductive organs," "seminal vesicle or womb," "seminal vessel" etc. I myself made the same mistake (1975). Later this mistake has been corrected: "Something must be said about the 'organ' bsam seẖu. This term does not appear in the text. Despite this the Tibetans regard this organ as one of the hollow organs (snod), the 6th in the group. It is possible that with the term bsam seẖu the Tibetans wanted to create their equivalent of the Chinese organ Triple-warmer =sanjiao."

E. Finckh "Foundations of Tibetan Medicine," Vol. II, 1985; 58.

(3) F. Meyer "GSO-BA RIG-PA," Paris, 1983; 155: The same and very good explanations concerning *bsam seẖu* and the suggestion not to translate this term.

5. Some authors described these finger tips. The conclusion: all solid organs (*don*) are palpated with the right side of the finger tip and all hollow organs (*snod*) are palpated with the left side of the finger tip.

   See: Nagwang Dagpa:

   "La sphygmologie tibétaine." In: *Les Médecines Traditionelles de l'Asie.* Strasbourg 1981; 29.

6. This book was published in Beijing (1985), 319 pages. "Medical Investigation of Lunar King" was compiled around 720-740, about half a century earlier than the rGyud bźi." Cai Jingfeng, ICANAS 1986, "Towards the early development of Tibetan Medicine."

7. J. Ross (see Bibliography) points out (page 215) that there are five zang: *Shen, Pi, Gan, Xin and Fei*; and not in terms

of the six *zang*, since *Xin Bao* is included with *Xin*. This author writes that "Western schools of acupuncture used to teach that there are two depths, superficial and deep, corresponding to *Fu* and *Zang* respectively. But the Chinese approach to pulse-taking also includes a very different approach to depth, involving three depths: superficial, middle and deep..."

Bibliography

(A) *Tibetan Pulsology*—Western languages

Donden, Yeshi. *Pulse Diagnosis in Tibetan Medicine.* Tibetan Medicine Series No. 1; 13-19. Library of Tibetan Works and Archives, Dharamsala, 1980.

Finckh, Elisabeth. *Foundations of Tibetan Medicine.* Vol. II; 51-59. Robinson Books, London 1985.

Meyer, Fernand. *GSO-BA RIG-PA, Le système médical tibétain*, 152-157. Centre National de la Recherche Scientifique, Paris, 1983.

Ragpay, Lobsang. *Pulse Analysis in Tibetan Medicine.* Tibetan Medicine Series No. 3; 45-52. Library of Tibetan Works and Archives, Dharamsala, 1981.

Rechung Rinpoche. *Tibetan Medicine*, 93-96. London 1973.

Tsarong, T. J., transl. and ed. *Fundamentals of Tibetan Medicine*, 18-28. Tibetan Medical Centre, Dharamsala, 1981.

(B) *Chinese Pulsology*

I Classic books

Huang-ti Nei ching Su Wen (chapters 17-19)

Huang-ti Nei-ching Ling-Shu (chapters 5 and 17)

Veith, I. *The Yellow Emperor's Classic of Internal Medicine.* Univ. of California Press, Berkeley, 1972.

Mo-ching (Wang-Shu-ho; 265-316). *Mo-ching* is said to have been translated into Tibetan as early as medieval times.

Huard, P. and Ming Wong. *Chinesische Medizin.* Fischer paperback, 1973; 22.

Nan-ching. A classic pulsology book. Unschuld, P. U., trans. and annot. *Nan-Ching. The classic of difficult issues.* Berkeley, 1987.

II Western books

Kaptchuk, T. J. *Chinese Medicine: The Web that has no Weaver.* Rider, London, 1986.

Ross, J., *Zang Fu.* Churchill Livingstone, Edinburgh/London, 1985.

Porkert, M. *Lehrbuch der chinesischen Diagnostik.* Verlag fur Medizin, Heidelberg, 1976.

Characteristics of Pharmacology

GENERAL COMMENTS

Tibet, a country rich in minerals and plants, imported specific plants, such as ginseng from Korea, and many others from neighboring countries whilst itself exporting items like musk, borax etc.

The medicaments were collected on large or small expeditions according to specific rules. While the expeditions were in progress, young doctors received exact instructions regarding the plants, minerals etc. Normally, fruits were gathered in autumn and leaves in summer, branches were cut in spring and roots dug up in winter.

The preparation of the plants takes place in the "medicine house" (*sman khaṅ*) =pharmacy. After a very long and complicated working operation, the plants are pulverized before being made into liquids, pills, powders or pastes. Finally, the liquid medicaments are poured into small jars and the pills and powders wrapped in paper and inscribed accordingly.

The substance in which the medicine is taken plays an important role and is known as the "medicine horse" (*sman rta*). This may be water, sugar or honey.

Medicaments are administered individually, mostly in the morning and in the evenings. The finished medicaments themselves may contain up to thirty or forty different components. The composition of the medicaments and the preparations of the recipes are so multifarious that their enumeration would fill volumes. The wealth of experience which the Tibetan doctors have allows them to vary the composition of the medicaments according to the needs of an individual.

BOOKS

A very large part of Tibetan medical literature is concerned with medicaments and pharmacology, but, unfortunately, not one single book has been translated into Western languages. W. A. Unkrig—one of the leading experts of this field— points out that it is very difficult to determine the botanical, Latin equivalents of these Tibetan medicaments.

Right at the start of research into Tibetan medicine it is vital to determine the medical terminology from sources available. The most important pharmaceutical books were written by the Tibetan doctor bsTan ḫ́jin phun *chogs. He wrote several highly esteemed medical works (18th century). These books are also of such particular value because they were printed in the monastery of sDe dge. The blockprints from this monastery are considered to be particularly reliable.

The books:

1. *dri med śel goṅ (abbreviated title).*

The full title:

bdud nad gźom paḫi gñen po rći sman gyi nus pa rkyaṅ bśad gsal ston dri med śel goṅ

2. *dri med śel phreṅ* (abbreviated title).

The full title:

bdud rći sman gyi nus miṅ rnam par bśad pa dri med śel phreṅ

3. *lag len gces bsdus*

The *rGyud bźi* (Four Treatises) must be the starting point for any study. From the texts we learn that the pharmacology is described in the following chapters:

part II, chapters 19, 20 and 21
part IV, chapters 3-19

In this short paper the main aspects of the large field of Tibetan pharmacology— classification, taste, potency and preparations of medicaments—are to be described, following the texts of the *rGyud bźi*, with special reference to the Tibetan doctrine of the three-part division: wind, bile and phlegm.

CLASSIFICATION

The text (T II 20^{38-40})

rin po che yi sman daṅ sa rdoḫi sman //
śiṅ sman rći sman thaṅ sman sṅo sman daṅ //
srog chags sman daṅ dbye ba brgyad du bśad //

This is the classic division into eight parts:
I Precious medicines (*rin po che yi sman*) (gems and metals)
II Medicinal earths (*sa yi sman*)
III Medicinal (substances obtained from) stones (*rdo sman*)
IV Medicinal (substances obtained from) trees (*śiṅ sman*)
V Medicinal essences, fluids (of a certain mucilaginous consistency) (*rći sman*)
VI Medicinal potions? Syrups? (unclear definition) (*thaṅ sman*)
VII Medicinal plants (roots, leaves, flowers) (*sṅo sman*)
IIX Medicines from sentient creatures (*srog chags sman*).

TASTE

The text (T II 19^{12-13})

sa chu me sa chu me chu daṅ rluṅ //
me rluṅ sa rluṅ gñis kyis ro drug skyed //

earth-water, fire-earth, water-fire, water and wind,
fire-wind, earth-wind: (the elements taken two)
by two produce six tastes.

This means: the types of taste (*ro*) result from the effects of the elements, from the interaction of two elements as follows:

earth and water=sweet
fire and earth=sour
water and fire=saline
water and wind=bitter
fire and wind=pungent
earth and wind=astringent

The five elements are: earth (*sa*), water (*chu*), fire (*me*), wind (*rluṅ*), ether (*mkhaḫ*). The element ether penetrates all medicaments.

The assignment of the tastes to the three humors is as follows: The text (T II 19[67-69])

mṅar skyur lan ćha ćha bas rluṅ ḫjoms śiṅ //
kha daṅ mṅar daṅ bska bas mkhris pa sel //
ćha skyur lan ćhas bad kan sel bar byed //

Sweet, sour, saline, pungent overcome wind,
bitter and sweet and astringent remove bile,
pungent, sour, saline remove phlegm.

The six tastes are assigned to wind, bile and phlegm as follows:

wind	bile	phlegm
sweet (mṅar)	bitter (kha)	pungent (ćha)
sour (skyur)	sweet (mṅar)	sour (skyur)
saline (lan ćha) pungent (ćha)	astringent (bska)	saline (lan ćha)

The *sweet* taste:

useful for old people and children, for healing wounds and for generally strengthening the body; it brings long life. e.g. honey, meat, saffron, asparagus, etc.

The *sour* taste:

stimulates the digestion and the appetite.

e.g. figs, emblic myrobalan, buttermilk, curds, pomegranates, etc.

The *saline* taste:

stiff body, lack of appetite.

e.g. alum, rock salt, soda, horn salt, etc.

The *bitter* taste:

strengthens the memory, is good to counteract thirst, poisoning and fever.

e.g. gentian, figs, musk, barberry, etc.

The *pungent* taste:

useful in case of swellings, skin diseases, dropsy and wounds.

e.g. black pepper, onions, garlic, etc.

The *astringent* taste:

cleanses the skin, heals wounds.

e.g. sandal, tamarisk, beleric myrbalan, chebulic myrobalan etc.

POTENCY

Potency (*nus pa*) is "the effect of a medicine in the stomach" (H. A. Jäschke, *Dictionary*, p. 306).

"Potency is the power by which an action takes place" (*Caraka-Saṃhitā*, p. 171, 172).

The text (T II $20^{4\text{-}10}$)

nus pa lci snum bsil daṅ rtul ba daṅ //
yaṅ rćub ćha daṅ rno ba rnam pa brgyad //
daṅ po bźi pos rluṅ daṅ mkhris pa sel //
ḫog ma bźi yis bad kan sel bar byed //
yaṅ rćub bsil ba gsum gyis rluṅ skyed ciṅ //
ćha rno snum pa gsum gyis mkhris pa skyed //
lci snum bsil rtul bźi yis bad kan skyed //

Heavy, oily, cool and dull and
light, rough, hot and sharp are the eight potencies.
The first four of them remove wind and bile.
The last four of them remove phlegm.
Light, rough, cool: these three produce wind.
Hot, sharp, oily: these three produce bile.
Heavy, oily, cool, dull: these four produce phlegm.

The eight potencies are: (1) heavy (*lci*); (2) oily (*snum*); (3) cool (*bsil*); (4) dull (*rtul*); (5) light (*yaṅ*); (6) rough (*rćub*); (7) hot (*ćha*); (8) sharp (*rno*).

Removing diseases:
heavy (*lci*), oily (*snum*)—wind
cool (*bsil*), dull (*rtul*)—bile
light (*yaṅ*), rough (*rćub*), hot (*ćha*), sharp (*rno*)—phlegm.

Producing diseases:
light (*yaṅ*), rough (*rćub*), cool (*bsil*)—wind
hot (*ćha*), sharp (*rno*), oily (*snum*)—bile
heavy (*lci*), oily (*snum*), cool (*bsil*), dull (*rtul*)—phlegm.

We see the following opposites:
heavy-light; oily-rough; cool-hot; dull-sharp;
light-heavy; rough-oily; hot-cool; sharp-dull.

The eight potencies are assigned to wind, bile and phlegm as follows:

wind	bile	phlegm
heavy (*lci*)	cool (*bsil*)	light (*yaṅ*)
oily (*snum*)	dull (*rtul*)	rough (*rćub*)
		hot (*ćha*)
		sharp (*rno*)

There are some discrepancies between these terms and those which are to be found in the system (T I 5^{18-20}): wind: smooth (*ḥjam*); bile: thin (*sla*); phlegm: hot (*ćha*).

PREPARATIONS

The text (T I 5[21-32])

ro nus de la sbyor ba źi sbyaṅ gñis //
źi byed rluṅ la khu ba sman mar gñis //
mkhris paḫi nad la thaṅ daṅ cur nis bsten //
bad kan nad la ril bu tres sam sbyar //

In relation to those tastes and potencies there are two (kinds of) preparations: (making) calm (and making) clean.

(As for those that) make calm, in the case of wind, there are two (kinds): soups (and) medicinal oils.

In the case of bile diseases one must take syrups and powders.

One must prepare pills (and) pastes in the case of phlegm.

khu ba rus khu bcud bźi mgo khrol te //
sman mar jā ti sgog skya ḫbras bu gsum //
rća ba lṅa daṅ sman chen dag la sbyar //
ma nu sle tres tig ta ḫbras buḫi thaṅ //
ga bur ćan dan gur gum cu gaṅ phye //
bćan dug ćhva sna rnams kyi ril bu daṅ //
tres sam se ḫbru da lis rgod ma kha //
ćhva daṅ coṅ źi bsregs paḫi thal sman no //

The following eight preparations *calm wind diseases*:
Soups (*khu ba*):
soups from bones (*rus khu*), the four juices (*bcud bźi*) *"mgo khrol"* (old and ground sheep's head soup).
Medicinal oils (*sman mar*):
nard (*jā ti*), garlic (*sgog skya*), the three fruits (ḫbras bu gsum = the three myrobalans), the five roots (*rća ba lṅa*), aconites (*sman chen*).

The following eight preparations *calm bile diseases*:
Syrups (*thaṅ*):

orrisroot (*ma nu*), guduch (*sle tres*), chirata (*tig ta*), the three fruits (*ẖbras bu gsŭm*).
Powders (*cur ni*):
camphor (*ga bur*), sandal (*ćan dan*), saffron (*gur gum*), bamboo manna (*cu gaṅ*).

The following seven preparations *calm phlegm diseases*:
Pills (*ril bu*):
aconites (*bćan dug*) various kinds of salt (*ćhva sna rnams*).
Pastes (*tres sam*):
pomegranates (*se ẖbru*), rhododendrons (*da li*), "mare face" (*rgod ma kha* = a preparation of sharp substances), alkaline medicaments made from burnt salts (*ćhva bsregs paẖi thal sman*), white stone (*coṅ źi*).

The text (T I 5[33-37])

sbyoṅ byed rluṅ gi nad la ẖjam rći ste //
mkhris pa bśal la bad kan skyugs kyis sbyaṅ //
ẖjam rći sle ẖjam bkru ẖjam bkru ma slen //
bśal la spyi bśal sgos bśal drag daṅ ẖjam //
skyugs la drag skyugs ẖjam skyugs gñis su sbyar //

(As for those preparations that) make clean, (they are) in the case of wind disease: oily enemas. (In the case of) bile (disease): laxatives.
(In the case of) phlegm (disease they make) clean with emetics. Oily enemas: (one prepares) mild enemas, purgative enemas, purgatives that are not mild.
In the case of laxatives (one prepares): general laxatives, particular laxatives, severe and mild laxatives.
In the case of emetics: two (forms): severe and mild emetics.

The following three preparations *clean wind diseases*:
Oily enemas (*ẖjam rći*):
Mild (*sle ẖjam*), purgative (*bkru ẖjam*), purgative—not mild (*bkru ma slen*).

The following four preparations *clean bile diseases*:

Laxatives (*bśal sman*):
General (*spyi*), particular (*sgos*), severe (*drag*), mild (*ḫjam*).
The following two preparations *clean phlegm diseases*:
Emetics (*skyugs sman*):
Severe (*drag*), mild (*ḫjam*).

This is of course a very short description of the preparations: the chapters of the *rGyud bźi* with regard to this field are voluminous! But this description is of some advantage because all terms are derived from the Tibetan texts which fill many pages of this paper. Moreover, it is quite clear that in these passages not only the preparations, but also the taste and potency of the medicaments are related to the three-part division of Tibetan medicine.

SUMMARY:

A very large part of Tibetan medical literature is concerned with pharmacology. Of course it is impossible to present the large field of pharmacology in a short paper. The attempt has been made to present a general view, a description of the most important topics:
(1) Books: the highly esteemed medical works of bsTan ḫjin phun ćhogs.
(2) The standard work *rGyud bźi* must be the starting point for any study. Pharmacology is described: part II, chapters 19, 20, 21 and part IV, chapters 3-9. Right at the start it is vital to determine the medical terminology from this source. The terms of the most important topics are derived from these texts, preceding the translations.
(3) Classification (classic division into eight parts).
(4) Taste of the medicaments sweet, sour, saline, bitter, pungent and astringent=6.
(5) Potency of the medicaments heavy, oily, cool, dull, light, rough, hot and sharp=8.
(6) Preparations: It was possible to make quite clear, that in these passages not only the preparations but also the taste and

potency of the medicaments are related to the three-part division of Tibetan medicine.

This means that treatment is governed by the patient's constitution. It is obvious that without a recognition of the type, treatment is impossible.

The presentation of this paper should serve to broaden the theoretical foundations in a systematic way. Very careful examination of the rich store of Tibetan medicaments is necessary in order that the West may benefit from the precious Tibetan medicaments.

Constitutional Types

Right at the start of research into Tibetan medicine, it is vital to determine the medical terminology and the latter has to be taken from the sources. The starting-point is the standard work of the Tibetan doctors, the *rGyud bzhi* = Four Treatises. It is from the text of this book that we learn that the basic principle of Tibetan medicine is the three-part division. The three "humors" are wind (*rlung*), bile (*mkhris pa*) and phlegm (*bad kan*). Part 1 of the above-mentioned book also includes a description of the System of Tibetan medicine which is made up of three Roots:

Arrangement (Root A)	Diagnosis (Root B)	Therapy (Root C)
healthy organism (I)	observation (III)	nutrition (VI)
diseased organism (II)	palpation (IV)	behavior (VII)
	questioning (V)	medicines (VIII)
		treatments (IX)

These are the 9 Disciplines of Tibetan medicine which can be described by following the System (International Seminar on Tibetan Studies, Oxford, 1979). The System also served as a connecting thread throughout to show the connection between the three humors and the methods of treatment (Csoma de Kórös Symposium, Velm-Wien, 1981).

In this paper *all* the terms which have in the meantime been derived from the texts are summarized, again by following the System.

In order to add more color and clarity to the description of the three humors, mention is also made of characteristics which are to be found in the second part of the Four Treatises (I. nature and temper, II. conditions which give rise to diseases).

It follows that the three humors are, through diagnostic methods, recognized as *types* to which specific kinds of treatment are assigned so that one can speak of a doctrine of constitution.

THE WIND-TYPE

I Nature and Temper.[1] Small, graceful, dark-skinned, sensitive to cold, talkative, lively, communicative, likes to laugh and sing; bad sleeper; span of life is short; characteristics are similar to those of the vulture, the raven and the fox.

II Conditions which give rise to disease.[2] Dissolute life, lack of sleep, sleepless nights, hard work, long conversations when hungry, vehement crying, frequent vomiting, losses of blood; worry and sorrow.

III Characteristics. *Root A* = Arrangement (of the parts of the body).

Trunk I = Healthy organism. Sustaining life, moving upwards, penetrating, (accompanying) fire, removing downwards.

Trunk II = Diseased organism. Producing (primary) cause = passion; produces 42 illnesses. Site (of diseases caused by wind) = lower part of the body. The 5 paths of circulation along which wind disorders arise: 1) Constituents of the body = bones. 2) Impurities = [little hairs of the skin], [touch]. 3) Sensory organs = ears [touch]. 4) Solid organs = heart [life-veins]. 5) Hollow organ = large intestine. Age = an old person suffers mainly from wind diseases. Place = in fragrant-windy and cold regions wind diseases predominate. Time =

in the rainy season (summer), in early evening (afternoon) and at dawn wind diseases occur.

Root B = Diagnosis.

Trunk III = Observation. Tongue (of a person suffering from wind diseases) = red, dry and rough. Urine (of a person suffering from wind diseases) = like water and has big bubbles.

Trunk IV = Palpation. Pulse (of a person suffering from wind diseases) = swimming, empty and stopping at times.

Trunk V = Questioning. 1) (Productive) causes = affected by *light and rough* food and behavior? 2) Conditions of illness = gaping and shuddering? stretching? shivering with cold? pain in all (bone) joints of the thigh and the hip? indefinite aches that change? vomiting on an empty stomach? whether the sense organs are bright; whether knowledge is stifled; pains when the patient is hungry? If these symptoms are present, the patient is a wind-type and is suffering from a wind disease. 3) Food = whether the patient feels better after eating food which is *oily*.

Root C = Therapy

Trunk VI = Nutrition. 1) Food = Horse (flesh), donkey (flesh), marmot (flesh), flesh that is a year old, śa chen, sesame oil, oil that is a year old, crude sugar, garlic, onions. 2) Drink = milk, carrot and onion soup, liquid (extract of) crude sugar, bone-soup.

Trunk VII = Behavior. To keep agreeable company. To have a warm place.

Trunk VIII = Medicines. 1) Taste = sweet, sour and saline (preferred tastes for wind-medicines). 2) Potency = oily, heavy and smooth (preferred potencies for wind-medicines). 3) Preparations that make calm = a) Soups = soup from bones, the four juices, mgo khrol. b) Medicinal oils = nard, garlic, the three fruits, the five roots, aconites. 4) Preparations that make clean = Oily enemas = mild, purgative and purgative—not mild.

Trunk IX = Treatments (external). 1) Inunction with massage; 2) Mongolian cauterization.

THE BILE-TYPE

I Nature and temper. Medium sized, yellowish color of the skin, cannot endure hunger and thirst well, sweats easily and a great deal; is talented and proud; span of life is of average length; characteristics are similar to those of the tiger and the ape.

II Conditions which give rise to disease. Sleeping during the afternoon, excessive strain when lifting heavy objects, too much movement in every respect— especially when the weather is warm. Annoyance.

III Characteristics *Root A* = Arrangement (of the parts of the body)

Trunk I = Healthy organism. Causing digestion, producing brightness (of chyle), satisfying (desires), (causing) vision, (making) clear the color (of the skin).

Trunk II = Diseased organism. Producing (primary) cause = hate; produces 26 diseases. Site (of diseases caused by bile) = middle part of the body. The 5 paths circulation along which bile disorders arise: 1) Constituent of the body = blood. 2) Impurity = sweat. 3) Sensory organ = eye. 4) solid organ = liver. 5) Hollow organs = gallbladder, small intestine. Age = a young person suffers mainly from bile diseases. Place = in dry and hot regions bile diseases predominate. Time = in the autumn, at noon and at midnight bile diseases occur.

Root B = Diagnosis.

Trunk III = Observation. Tongue (of a person suffering from bile diseases) = covered with thick, tawny phlegm. Urine (of a person suffering from bile diseases) = reddish-yellow, much vapor, hot smell.

Trunk IV = Palpation. Pulse (of a person suffering from bile diseases) = beats quickly, strongly and subtly.

Trunk V = Questioning. 1) (Productive) causes = affected by *sharp and hot* food and behavior? 2) Conditions of illness = bitter taste? fever (hot flesh)? aches in the upper part (of the body)? pains after digestion? If these symptoms are present, the patient is a bile-type and is suffering from a bile disease. 3) Food = whether the patient feels better after eating food which is cool.

Root C = Therapy.

Trunk VI = Nutrition. 1) Food = Curds of cow and goat, buttermilk, fresh butter, game-flesh, goat-flesh, fresh flesh of animals of mixed breed, young barley, skyabs, dandelions. 2) Drink = hot water, cool water, boiled and cooled water.

Trunk VII = Behavior. Sit calmly. Have a cool place.

Trunk VIII = Medicines. 1) Taste = sweet, bitter and astringent (preferred tastes for bile-medicines); 2) Potency = cool, thin and blunt (preferred potencies for bile medicines); 3) Preparations that make calm = a) Syrups = orrisroot, guduchi, chirata, the three fruits; b) Powders = camphor, sandal, saffron, bamboo manna. 4) Preparations that make clean = Laxatives = general, particular and severe laxatives.

Trunk IX = Treatments (external) 1) Production of sweat; 2) Blood-letting; 3) The magic water-wheel.

THE PHLEGM-TYPE

I Nature and temper. Plump and tall, pale-skinned, cool body; can endure hunger and thirst well, deep sleeper, pleasant and friendly disposition; his span of life is long; his characteristics are similar to those of the lion and bell-wether.

II Conditions which give rise to disease. Sleeping during the day, rest after meals, staying in damp regions, bathing for too long, too light clothing, eating too much and too quickly.

III Characteristics *Root A* = Arrangement (of the parts of the body).

Trunk I = Healthy organism. Supporting, decomposing, (causing) taste, (causing) satisfaction, causing to bind (the joints together).

Trunk II = Diseased organism. Producing (primary) cause = delusion; produces 33 diseases. Site (of diseases caused by phlegm) = upper part of the body. The 5 paths of circulation along which phlegm disorders arise: 1) Constituents of the body

= chyle, flesh, fat, marrow and semen. 2) Impurities = faeces and urine. 3) Sensory organs = nose and tongue. 4) solid organs = spleen, kidneys and lungs. 5) Hollow organs = stomach, urinary-bladder.

Root B = Diagnosis.

Trunk III = Observation. Tongue (of a person suffering from phlegm diseases) = gray, thick, lustreless, smooth and moist. Urine (of a person suffering from phlegm diseases) = white, little odor, little vapor.

Trunk IV = Palpation. Pulse (of a person suffering from phlegm diseases) = sinking, weak and slow.

Trunk V = Questioning. 1) (Productive) causes = affected by *heavy and oily* food and behavior? 2) Conditions of illness = uncomfortable appetite? difficulty in digesting food? vomiting? (bad taste) in the hollow of the mouth? distended stomach? eructation? whether body and mind are heavy (together)? cold both inside and outside? discomfort after eating? If these symptoms are present, the patient is a phlegm-type and is suffering from a phlegm disease. 3) Food = whether the patient feels better after eating food which is *warm.*

Root C=Therapy.

Trunk VI = Nutrition. 1) Food = sheep (flesh), wild yak (flesh), beasts of prey (flesh), fish-flesh, honey, hot pap of old grain from dry land. 2) Drink = curds and buttermilk of the yak, strong beer, boiled water.

Trunk VII = Behavior. Take an energetic walk. Have a warm place.

Trunk VIII = Medicines. 1) Taste = pungent, sour and astringent (preferred tastes for phlegm-medicines); 2) Potency = sharp, rough and light (preferred potencies for phlegm-medicines); 3) Preparations that make calm = a) Pills = aconite, various kinds of salt; b) Pastes = pomegranates, rhododendrons, mare face, alkaline medicaments (made) from burnt salt, white stone. 4) Preparations that make clean = emetics. Severe and mild emetics.

Trunk IX = Treatments (external). 1) Heat treatments; 2) Cauterization.

This systematic summary (which still does not include all the characteristics of the three types—in the book *Four Treatises* many more are mentioned) does, however, show just how clearly the three types are set out. Nevertheless, in practice the three types do not always occur in such an unadulterated form—more often one finds mixed types. It is a well-known fact that Western medicine is also aware of a large number of divisions into constitutional types and here, too, there are very many mixed types which are often very difficult to diagnose.

The Tibetans categorize their mixed types according to a very simple method—a distinction is made between 7 kinds: 1) the pure wind, bile, and phlegm types = 3 kinds; 2) one type displaying the characteristics of all three types = 1 kind; 3) the types with pairs of characteristics: wind + bile, wind + phlegm, bile + phlegm = 3 kinds.

It is not the task of this paper to differentiate the characteristics of the three types which have been mentioned with regard to the influences upon them, i.e. Indian, Chinese etc. Nor can the typically Tibetan features be mentioned here such as the anamnesis with its 29 questions, the exact assignment of food and drink and the assignment of the methods of treatment to the three humors.

On the contrary, the purpose of this paper is to point out quite clearly that it is only be means of the precisely-defined diagnostic methods that the respective types with their symptoms of illness can be recognized and that successful treatment is only possible if the method of treatment assigned to this type is applied.

NOTES

1. *rGyud bzhi*, Part 2, Chapter 6.
2. *rGyud bzhi*, Part 2, Chapter 9.

This paper was first published in *American Journal of Chinese Medicine*, Vol. XII, Nos. 1-4 (1984), pp. 44-49, by the Institute for Advanced Research in Asian Science and Medicine, New York.

Transliteration

Chapters 1 and 5

ka	kha	ga	nga
ca	cha	ja	nya
ta	tha	da	na
pa	pha	ba	ma
tza	tsha	dza	wa
zha	za	’a	ya
ra	la	sha	sa
ha	a		

Chapters 2, 3 and 4:

ka	kha	ga	ṅ
ca	cha	ja	ña
ta	tha	da	na
pa	pha	ba	ma
ća	ćha	ǰa	
wa	źa	za	ẖa
ya	ra	la	
śa	sa	ha	a

Bibliography

Extensive bibliographies on Tibetan medicine:

(1) Clifford, Terry. *Tibetan Buddhist Medicine and Psychiatry.* Samuel Wieser, York Beach, 1984.

(2) Donden, Yeshi. *Health through Balance.* Snow Lion Publications, Ithaca, New York, 1986.

(3) Finckh, Elisabeth. "Grundlagen tibetischer Heilkunde." Vol. I ML Uelzen 1975; Vol. II. ML Uelzen 1985. *Foundations of Tibetan Medicine.* Vol. I, Watkins Publishing, London, 1978; Vol. II, Robinson Books, London, 1985. 2nd edition 1987.

(4) Meyer, Fernand. *GSO-BA RIG-PA. Le système médical tibétain.* Centre National de la Recherche Scientifique, Paris, 1983.

(5) Rechung Rinpoche. *Tibetan Medicine.* Wellcome Institute of the History of Medicine, London, 1973. California Press, Berkeley, 1976.

(6) Tsarong, T.J. (trans. and ed.). *Fundamentals of Tibetan Medicine.* Tibetan Medical Centre, Dharamsala, 1981.